Filipina Girls

and the

Dark Art of *Seduction*

Content

"Make money in the first world and make love in the third world."

- Anonymous.

Foreword

It's no great secret that a man needs no game to win pretty women here in the Philippines. Any expat will tell you this. Just show up, crack a joke and these cute Pinays will beg you to be the father of their kids. All by the second date.

Seven years ago it was a different story for me. I lived in Toronto, though 'lived' seems far too tame a word. Survived is more like it.

Toronto, or Dark Elf City as many men now call it, is straight out of a Drow fantasy novel. You don't want to visit such a place. It's a dark, dreary place where matriarchal women shun eye contact, dye their hair like punk rockers and punish (severely I might add) nice guy efforts like opening doors, compliments or just being an all-around gentleman.

Not all of them mind you, *but most of them.*

On a good day, a woman may only walk across the street to avoid you. On a bad day...

- You get screamed at for wanting to drive her car.

- Horsewhipped if you root for 'Him' in a major divorce court proceeding.

- Shanked for flashing a look of disapproval on her new blue-green hair.

This brutal dating scene grew so depressing that I began to wonder if a few of these women, like the Drow of the Underdark, preferred to eat animals that were still living because they believed the meat had a better flavor. Was I next on the menu?

Yes indeed. I discovered my fiancée had been banging an Italian for three months in my own kitchen. It seemed she disapproved of my desire to wait 6 months before marriage and this was her way of letting her 'feelings' air out.

My self-confidence destroyed, I thought of jumping off the CN Tower but my fear of great heights kept me grounded. It didn't stop there. I tried other ways but chickened out. I didn't know it at the time, but someone else quite close to me would give me a good shove into the high air - my dad. I have been flying high ever since he intervened.

My dad, the biggest penny-pincher on planet Earth, the man who bought me Hot Wheels for my 18th birthday, had just given me a $1200 ticket to Cebu, Philippines as a way out of this horrifically dark past, present and future. The man who just spent a small fortune on my misfortune. Why this? Why now?

Well as luck would have it, boarding that flight turned out to be the best decision of my life. You will find out as I did that Filipinas know how to make a man feel like a King. An Emperor.

In fact, as soon as I got off the plane, I felt the difference in the very air. I looked up and the neck strain was gone. It was as though the noose that had been swaying over my head for years - put there by feminist Toronto girls - had been pulled away. Years, *years* of abuse began to heal as a result of meeting Asian girls in Cebu, Davao and Makati. I had found the cure for cancer in the West: The Far East!

Here, as in Thailand, they approach <u>you</u> *and not the other way around.* That was the first shocker. The second was that girls came as varied as pebbles on a beach - and you will have your pick of them all.

Spanish-Cebuanas
Half-Chinese minxes
Polynesian Fire-Twirling Filipinas

They come in every form you can imagine:

Real estate agents. Secretaries. Models. Beauty contestants. Beach fire-dancers. Casino Blackjack dealers. Teachers. Tutors. All of them want to give you that 'girlfriend experience' you last experienced as a teenager.

Too old? They could care less. It isn't in their vocabulary. They *prefer* older men.

Listen. Girls just want a nice guy who won't blackjack them senseless and make them look bad in front of their friends. That's all. Just a guy who'll show em a good time and smile. They don't want the Fifty Shades guy. They don't even want a 'bad boy' guy with a Harley and rap sheet a mile long. That card fails on every level here because

Heaven knows there are enough Pinoys that fit that bill to a tee.

Just Be a Nice Guy and it'll bring hot and wet rewards just as they do in Russia, Brazil, Columbia and Thailand.

To this end, I will teach you what other seduction books do not.

Most books on Filipinas will tell you how to bag the 5's and 6's, how to approach them in the malls, give out your number and hope they don't flake.

This book isn't about getting 5's and 6's.

It's about getting the 8's and 9's.

You didn't fly all the way around the world to make love to 5's did you? Right. You can get that any day of the week. You flew over here to get what you couldn't back home: a smoking-hot girl who is way out of your league.

I will teach you all I know in this regard.

Chapter 1: Super Pipelining

Before we go into the various pros and cons of the major dating sites, we need to first define what pipelining is, and how you oh intrepid adventurer can utilize it to slay young pussy.

So what is pipelining? It's when you hit up several girls a month before your flight, or maybe 3 weeks prior with the intent to weed out the time-wasters. The point is to not have all your ducks in a row. Your ducks are spread out with no one central point of failure.

Below: a pipeline schematic of a microprocessor. Your brain works in much the same way.

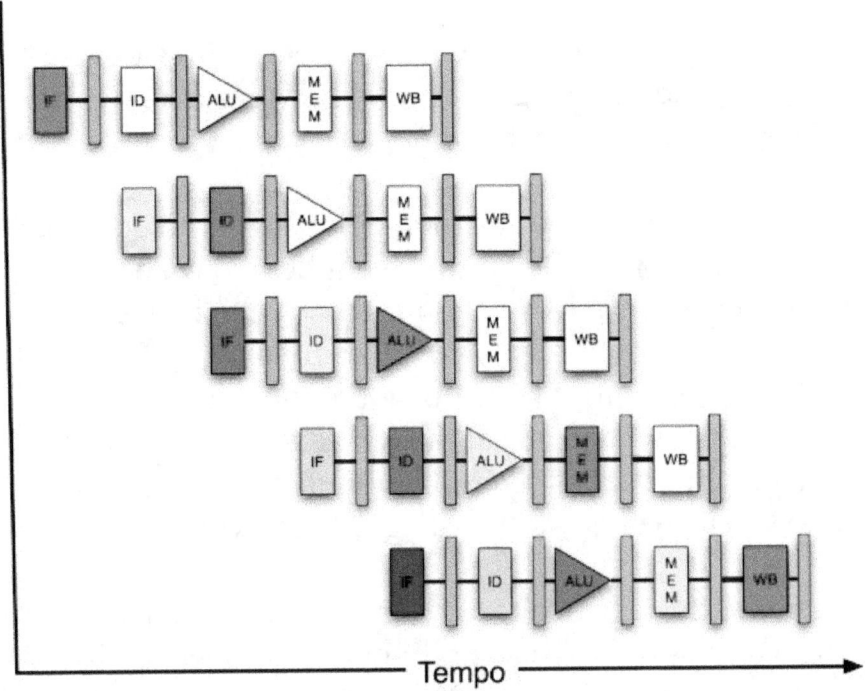

Tempo

"You get used to it. Your brain does the translating. I don't even see the code. All I see is blonde, brunette, redhead. Hey uh, you want a drink?" - Cypher, The Matrix

Believe it or not, your brain or more specifically, your <u>subconscious,</u> knows more about what's good for you then you do (*you* here being the front part of your brain). Redheads, brunettes, blondes, it's a game of push/pull, cat/mouse and pipelining is a great strategy that even poker players use to up their chances of scoring BIG either in Vegas or in Florida at the blackjack tables.

If done correctly it'll give you a safety net in case calamity happens - which often does.

Like if one girl decides to split your heart with a double-bladed axe and doesn't give two fig newtons about your feelings - you can ditch her more easily.

Not pipelining can be catastrophic. It's harder to do it that way as a newcomer. Better to have it be like water off a duck's back and the way we do that is by having several girls at our disposal. The *other girls* in your 'pipeline'. Having just one girl you've flown around the world to meet, and an average one at that, makes the experience much, much harder as she's likely to throw down a lot of drama when she knows she can get away with it.

Remember this above all: It is You who are the high value in most anyplace in Asia - Philippines, Indonesia, China, Thailand and esp. Vietnam. Not her. Even 9.5s are lightyears easier to get here than back home. But you need to know this going in or you will shoot too low and end up with a bland '5' when you could have gotten a '9'. The idea here is to get the best bang for your buck. Pipelines help you obtain this.

Good pipelining requires a half-decent poker face as it's little like spinning plates. That is, you try to keep the plates spinning so that no one plate falls to the floor due to lack of motion.

For example: You buy five plates and paint each plate with a girl's face and a number depicting their place on your personal preference scale. Beauty. Sex appeal. Legs. Tits. Whatever floats your boat.

Take a moment to close your eyes and imagine spinning this plates all at once. A few plates spin faster than others. They'll last the longest while a few will fall to the floor and shatter. Some faces on the plates have girl's with an acute acne problem. Another has height disadvantage since she's 4'9. Still another has 2 kids.

Some of these girls (plates) want to move way way faster than the others. They're hitting you up for marriage before you've even met them and most of the time it's because they view you as a white ATM. They're asking you to send money. A few are even hitting you up for sex via webcam in order to blackmail you on Facebook if you don't pay up. Truthfully, you needn't do any of this.

All you need to do is Keep Her Interested until you fly in. That's it.

- Do not send money. Ever. No matter what she does.
- Do not give in to fake tears.
- Do not care about her 'sick cow' and ridiculous claims that the entire family will starve unless you buy her cow some medicine. It's all tits on a bull.

Many Filipinas have the attention span of a moth. For this reason I don't recommend hitting up any dating site for more than 3 weeks prior to touchdown since many will find someone else or just plain forget who you are.

Filipinas live in the here and now and this is their Achilles Heel - one we will use to our advantage because, if you pipeline a woman for 3 months, she'll be expecting a ring on your finger when you land. Things move that fast here and anything past 3 weeks flies right into the danger zone

Points to Note:

Limited Visit - Be vague about how long you are staying. Some countries, such as Latin America, girls lose interest if they discover you're only going to be around for 2 weeks. It's the same in the Philippines. Girls get a whiff that you're just a tourist passing through and they lose interest. So get a business card online with your email and tell them 6 months at the least. A year is better. Travel writer. Real estate. Restaurant scout. Whatever.

Beautiful Girls - Be careful with hitting up the most beautiful women on dating sites. They get 50 messages or more per day and many are p4p (pay for pussy) hookers. Get the 7's and up interested first since the upper echelon of women most probably will not give you the time of day. For 8's and above we will hit up the beauty contests (more on this in a bit) as it's all but guaranteed they will NOT be on the dating sites. That's because they do not need to.

Must Have Tools for Pipelining

Settling in

Google Maps - Know where you are at all times. Tondo, Zamboanga, downtown Manila at night = The Dead Zones.

Google Translate - A few stunners on FilipinaCupid did not speak the best English. This app helps with that, but also helps in cabs, hotels, markets & cafes.

Swiftkey - This app uses A.I. to predict the next word you intend to type, but you can also switch to a different language keyboard like Spanish or Italian to ease communication.

1-Click Tether - WiFi tethering; use it to get internet-connected on Windows, Mac, phone, tablet, Ubuntu, Wii, PS3 if the WiFi is terrible (or you experience a brownout. Happens often in the Phils!). Requires no root.

Pipelining

Badoo - An excellent all-around pipeline tool. Shows you the people nearby, and—the people you've bumped into in real life.

Tinder - Self-explanatory.

Fake GPS - Good for finding girls in the city you intend to visit. Bonus: survey where the hottest Filipinas are according to region.

Couchsurfing - Stay with locals instead of staying at hotels or hostels.

Messaging

Facebook - Many Pinays use this to check if you're seeing other girls. Reverse-image lookup also can be a date killer so never put any photos on your fake FB page that you put on the real one. Online notifier plugin will also tell you when a specific girl is online. However, consider FB dangerous. I had noticed that my Viber contacts were popping up as 'suggested friends' on my FB page.

Note: I never gave my ph. number to Facebook but they found it anyway because if said phone number is on a friend's phone and they consent to share their contact list, they'll discover you.

Whatsapp: Cheap texting app many Pinays use. They favor Viber however.

Viber: Most popular chat app in the Philippines.

Chapter 2: Dating Sites

You create your own universe as you go along.
– Winston Churchill

Have you ever seen Lucy swipe the ball away from poor Charlie Brown and the very next day he falls victim to the scam *again*? A few Filipinas are like that. One thirsty guy after another and many fools and their money are soon parted. Many fools, many monies. It's amazing how us guys loathe validation queens here in the West but do the very same thing when it comes to Asian girls - just with different girls.

Thirsty, gullible men get ensnared by all the coo and baby talk because they're used to Ice Queens back home who curse them for asking for the time. Filipina affection is an incurable addiction if you're new to SE Asia. Sometimes it goes too far and you end up robbed, beaten and broke.

In Davao (southern Mindanao region), a few rich Canadians wind up kidnapped on occasion and beheaded because the Canadian Parliament doesn't give into terrorist demands. Much like with the U.S, you get kidnapped, you're on your own.

So don't wave money around.

Don't wear 'bling', especially on Skype.

Use your wits and soak up knowledge BEFORE you go.

Most of girls see western guys as a golden ticket out and if this is your first time in the Phils that means you're thirsty and susceptible to falling for the first Asian chick who sucks you off without charging you. Girls here are masters at exploiting feminist-injured Western men. They think you're as dumb as Forrest Gump. After reading this chapter, you won't be.

Targeting 6's and 7's. Avoid 8's and up as she's likely getting tons of messages.

First up is **Cherry Blossoms**.

Price: $30 dollars per month or $119 per year. Not 'free' like DateinAsia but then you get what you pay for. By paying you cut scammers off at the pass and avoid legions of ladyboys that hang out at free sites.

Quality of Girls: Varies at any one time but 7-8 range is not uncommon. Lots of 20ish girls and even post-30 lookers that spell attraction for most men of any age. Not too many teens and what is there is very spread out from Cebu to Davao to Illigan. While you have the funds to see her, most provincial girls do not have the funds to see you if you are far away. 40 and above guys do well here.

Age:

Note that 98% of the girls here have NO age specific preference in their profiles, (though older is seen as more stable), but you will want to avoid single moms if you're looking for a relationship (Pinoy dads cause trouble and if she's separated she can rat you to the cops and have you arrested for 'adultery'). Nevertheless, in SM Malls I frequently see 50 year old men with 18 year olds. Usually if the guy is a slob and dressed poorly it means he is taking care of her family's money needs.

Front Page: First thing you will notice when you login is the 'Most Viewed Member' as well as the Best Rated Profile Pic. The men (whom you cannot see while logged in as a male) vote for the hottest women. I'd avoid these profiles as they are getting swarmed with messages from thirsty men the world over - many of whom are married men who have zero intentions of flying off to meet them. I'll show you how to target 9's in the next chapter.

Points to Note

Exploit the Search Feature!

Let it ride overnight. Seriously, it works. Most Filipinas I've found are too casual to use the search bar of Cherry Blossoms to find their mates. They simply can't be bothered. You're much better off staying logged in all night. Midnight here, 12 noon there. Sleep, yes, but leave your laptop on and logged in and wake up to dozens of 'Smiles' and 'Emails' from Filipinas wanting to meet you. This also cuts out the time wasters, non-English speakers and scammers as they are easier to identify.

What to watch out for:

- Pictures with 4-star hotel rooms (who was she banging there?).
- Yachts or other big boats in Boracay ($$$).
- Shoving her tits in your face (and everyone else's),
- requests for money

Use common sense. What you see in her profile is what every other guy sees but count on her skin being two shades darker when you actually meet due to her Photo editing skills.

Money: Say she contacts you to say she's caught Dengue fever and death awaits at her door. Send money now! Or else the Grim Reaper will come.

Tell her you will NOT send money to any girl you have not met in person. No exceptions. Hit the Report Abuse button any time a girl does this (save a screenshot if in Skype). If you do meetup and she brings ANYONE else along without asking your permission first... walk away. She's just looking for a free meal.

The exception here is the 18 year olds who more than likely won't be allowed to see you without a chaperone. More on how to get around this later.

Filipina Cupid

Price: $30 per month. You can browse for free however much like Cherry Blossoms, you cannot respond to emails without paying.

Quality of Girls: Same as CherryBlossoms.

Age: Roughly the same, though many more single moms I've found here than at CherryBlossoms. Age preferences were the same for most girls.

Scams: One dangerous scam involves a filipina asking you to Skype with her. It's always the same. Guy likes her profile pics. Guy emails her. Girl bounces him to Skype. They make small talk for a while before she starts to get naked. She shows her tits while making seductive eyes and finally goes spread eagle for him. Rather than ask for money outright, she asks for his Facebook info.

Watch out. Here there be dragons.

Most guys say yes. Here's my Facebook info. Next thing you know she is reading off your contact list and says if you don't wire some cash to her she's going to post that sex video you just had with her to everyone from your TaeKwonDo master to Uncle Leo.

The solution:

1.) Never send naked pics of yourself. Certainly not one with your face front and center.

2.) Be careful with texts as they can be copied/pasted to places you do not wish it. Once it is out there, it is out there forever.

3.) If you have zero intentions of inviting the girl into your family structure or social ladder then there's no good reason to tell her your real name. A nickname will do (hide the passport/wallet/DL).

Date in Asia

Date in Asia is free, true. But 'free' is often synonymous with 'A fool and his money are soon parted'.

Many seasoned Filipinas that hang out here can game you better than you think. Do not underestimate them. They've had years of practice and know which knobs to turn just as James Bond did when it came to gaming women into bed for Queen and country. Seriously, they're aces at the skin trade and have been gaming guys for a golden ticket out of the Phils for so long that they could be CIA agents by now.

Never forget they are trying to make you feel like a richer, sexier King than the next girl over.

Other problems with DiA:

Ladyboys

A few ladyboys at Cherry Blossoms messaged me, but their numbers paled in comparison to the LEGIONS that hang out at Date in Asia. So if you're going for notch counts and are only staying in Asia for a week and want to try DiA... then you need to screen <u>heavily</u> for ladyboys.

You do this by asking them outright. "Are you a ladyboy?"

Each and every time.

A few may get offended but that's no big deal. The real girls are probably drama queens anyway. At the very least, you will filter out the *ladyboy drama*; drama that is a whole other level of pain that often involves bouncers and policemen.

Ask outright and do not care at all about offending them. Better yet, make sure to ask if she was *born as a woman* and not *if she is a woman*. More than a few ladyboys actually believe they are women, balls and all.

Photoshopped Pictures

A filipina's fascination with white skin often goes too far, such as them photoshopping their pictures to look as pale as their mixed-lineage soap opera stars. A general rule of thumb is that, most times, she will look worse than her least attractive profile picture and may even have acne. So keep your expectations in check and be willing to 'hurt her feelings' if an ogre shows up with a hairy-legged Auntie in tow.

Just walk away. You are the prize.

Chapter 3: How to Seduce a Filipina Supermodel

Right now a few of you are thinking, 'Why not just skip the pipeline and ask any salesgirl at SM Mall out on a date?' You could indeed. It's almost too easy to hand out a cell number on a scrap of paper and be banging hello within the hour.

The only problem is, it's *hard* to pinpoint where the 8s and 9s are in the malls. They're packed to the gills with 5's and 6's... but is that what you really want? Did you plunk down $1200 for a flight halfway around the world to date average girls? What we're aiming for are ABOVE-AVERAGE girls. Girls in the 7-8 range at a minimum. There's a clever way to do this that doesn't involve walking the beat in every SM Mall you find.

Beauty Pageants

One crafty way to do this is by gaming Beauty Contestants. Can you just picture yourself with any of these luscious ladies? Most western men can't and it isn't due to their looks, status or money. It's to do with the lack of self-confidence that Western society has drilled into them. Western *women*, to be more precise.

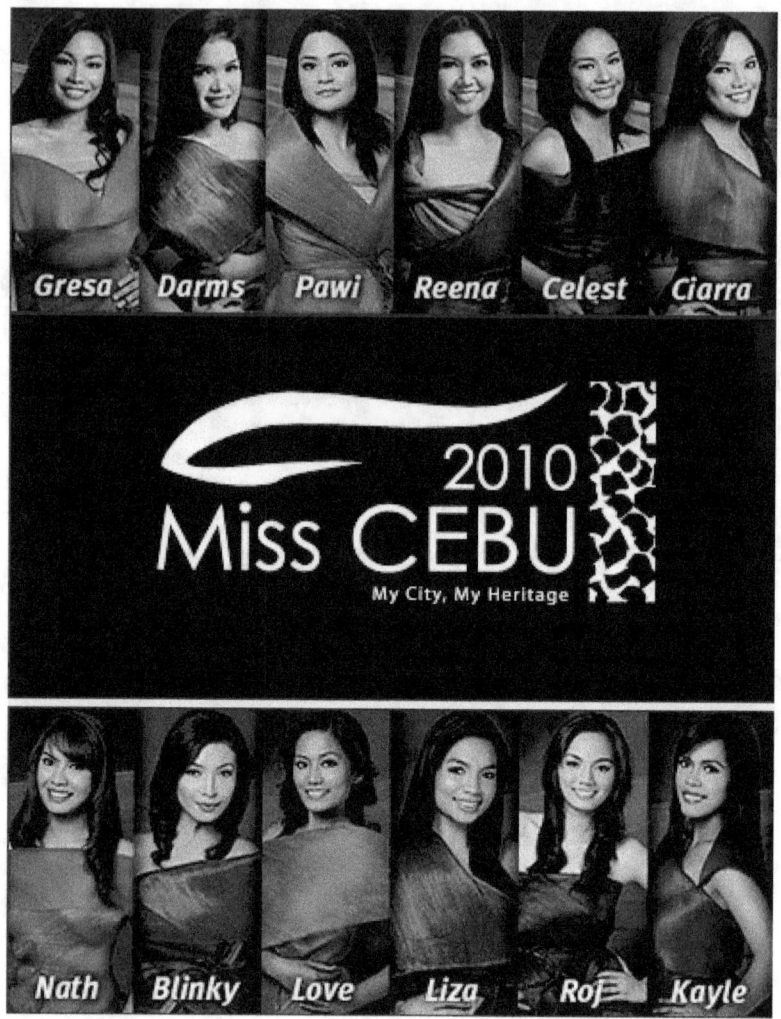

It's not exactly the most original idea since Pinoys have been gaming these fine fillies for far longer than us expats. But Filipina's view white-skinned Western men from the UK/USA/Canada with far less suspicion than your average Pinoy who shows up at one of these beauty holes intending on making her his diamond-worthy sex slave.

You are new meat to these girls. Good wholesome meat and rest assured that none of the above girls will be on any dating site. That's good for us as it cuts down competition by 90%. Plus, they will look at you like a princess would looking for a prince to sweep her away. That's why they are here.

You will bypass a lot of the fakers who photoshop their profile pictures to hide their acne (or kids), not to mention shortcut the high-society social circle game required to lay one of these 8's. To do so you have to go where the talent is, the same as you would in any major hub in the USA (Las Vegas, Manhattan or Montreal, Canada).

Since the Philippines has no Las Vegas equivalent, beauty pageants are the next best place as most casinos (Borocay) are plagued with hookers and scammers that prey on foreign thirsty men.

So our target are the pageants. All of em. The "Big Four" international pageants are Miss Universe, Miss World, Miss International and Miss Earth. The Philippines has won all of the Big Four titles, some more than once, but there are contests specific to Cebu and Manila and a few other places around the islands that many local Pinoys skip for one reason or another.

Recommended ones are:

1.) Miss Cebu

This one is held annually during the Sinulog Festival in January in Cebu, and is run by the city government.

2.) Binibining Pilipinas (correct spelling)

This pageant selects Filipina representatives in two of the Big Four international beauty pageants to compete in the Miss Universe contest.

3.) Miss Philippines Earth

Miss Philippines Earth is held annually in search of the most beautiful and environmentally-friendly woman in the Philippines. It is the largest and most widely participated beauty pageant in the Philippines with 50 ladies to choose from. (Fifty! Think about those odds for a moment)

4.) Miss Republic of the Philippines

This pageant was first staged in 1969. The Runners-up of Miss Republic were awarded as Miss Luzon (1st Runner-up), Miss Visayas (2nd Runner-up), Miss Mindanao (3rd Runner-up) and Miss Manila (4th Runner-up).

5.) Miss World Philippines

Miss World Philippines is the national franchise of the Miss World pageant in the Philippines and selects the country's representative to the said pageant.

Google the titles of any of these to get the times and dates as they change quite frequently.

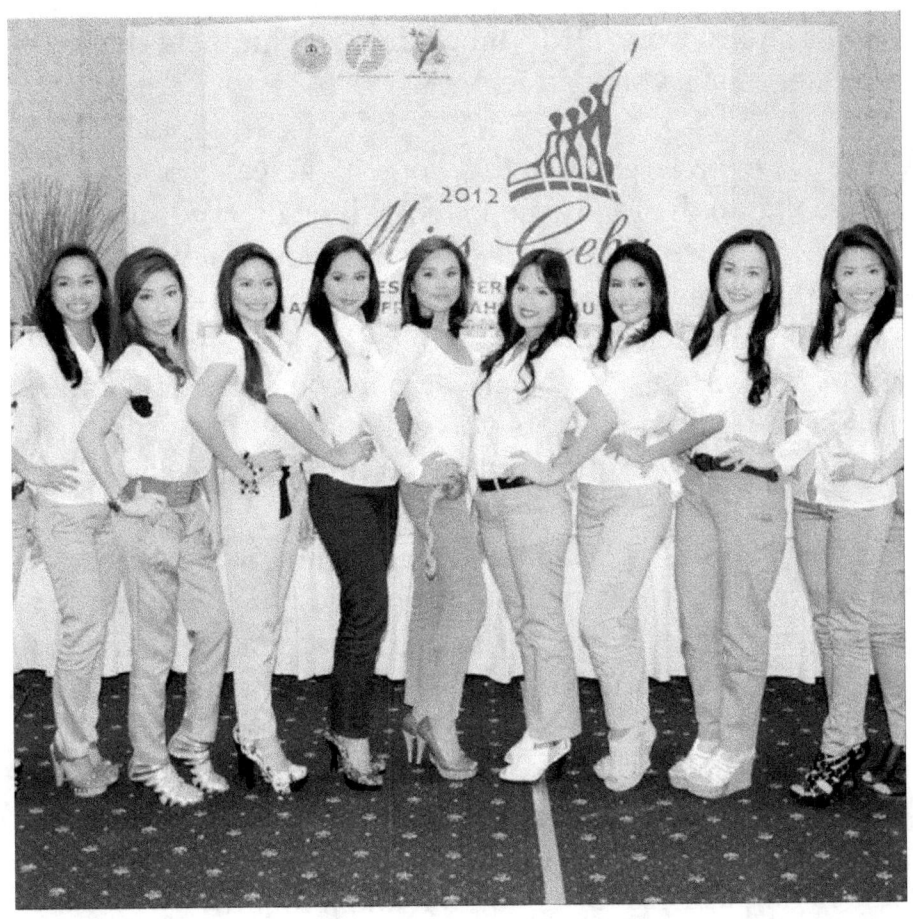

Strategy

Now then, for most of the pageants it is stupid easy to succeed. All you need to do is SHOW UP dressed for success.

75% of the Filipino men at these events are looking to marry off their daughters to the next John Wayne

Photographer from TIME magazine who hit them up in a nice suit (that's you, partner).

Rule 1: Do NOT gawk at the women - at least not initially. Leave that to the Pinoy men who will be there for that express purpose. Filipinas expect this though few want it. Want they want is stage recognition, a social ladder to something bigger. Filipinas are here because they are shrewd opportunists. You are here for business only and it will be the Filipino fathers you will talk to; the very same fathers of these beautiful nymphs in the pictures above.

Put business first, pleasure later. Just know your stuff. Photography. Real Estate. Investing. Tourism. Setting up a dive shop. Travel writer. Whatever. Just pick something you know a lot about (or even a little) and attend with confidence. An easy way to do this is by not giving a care what they think. This is not the USA. You will not be laughed at for wanting to start up a Great White Shark riding business... but you need to know something about it. A general business idea of vision and... money.

Rule 2: Do NOT blow off the fathers! I cannot stress this enough. Within 5 minutes of striking up a conversation, the daddies of the above beauties began to game me as a possible suitor for a lovely-yet-spoiled princess sweeter than any peach on Earth.

Keep your mouth shut for a few minutes to gauge his business expertise. Remember the Japanese story about two samurai meeting up in the rain? The first one to move loses the advantage. So keep your cool. You've done this before many times. The fathers here richly desire a successful foreigner in the family for when money is tight (among other things). You must seem successful to him without actually mentioning any numbers.

I left with 6 numbers of the hottest women you can imagine and all on my first time. That is, *after* I discovered it was wiser to engage the fathers in 'investment' talks then flirt with a woman who still has to introduce you to dear old dad. Game the father, hit two birds with one stone, and wake up smiling.

Downsides

Now for one annoying downside. With all that glamour and makeup and rock-hard tits and eyes that are to die for come the Princess Jasmine attitude. You may not see it at first glance. I sure didn't. But by the first date you'll see the bug-eyed, bushy-tailed squirrely hamster start peeking out. The beauty queen may not ask for money outright, but she may very well whip out a cell phone to answer an 'emergency' Viber message from her Aunty who wants to know the details on Mr. Bruce Wayne. The solution?

Call her on it. Tell her it's incredibly rude and lessens her stature to be a smartphone addict. If she persists then go full bore rich jerk game. You're a successful investor who owns a yacht, a fire pit and a winter cabin in Canada with a herd of rare elk and a ski lodge and a hot air balloon business. Why should you waste your time with her if she wants to blab all night to someone else?

Pretend to be thinking about something else, perhaps another Pageant girl, and glance at other women who stroll by. Don't gawk. Just comment on how pretty Ms. Davao was in the contest. If this fails then say something that displays your discomfort while letting out a small sigh. Something like,

"You know, I'd really like some good friends on my side here in the Phils. Maybe you could be one?"

She'll spot the 'friend-zone' attempt and either put the blasted cell away and focus on you or walk out. Either way you win.

Where to Take Your Beauty Girl

Now that you've got Jasmine's number, what next?

Take her someplace upscale, not *downscale*. This was another huge blunder of mine. I took my girl to the Cinema... big mistake. I looked like the biggest cheapskate in Asia and a moron to boot that didn't know squat about upper-class girl expectations. She cannot kiss you at the cinema without feeling awkward. She cannot talk without annoying the other cinema goers. To say nothing about riding you reverse-cowgirl and screaming your name. Instead, take her to...

Brique

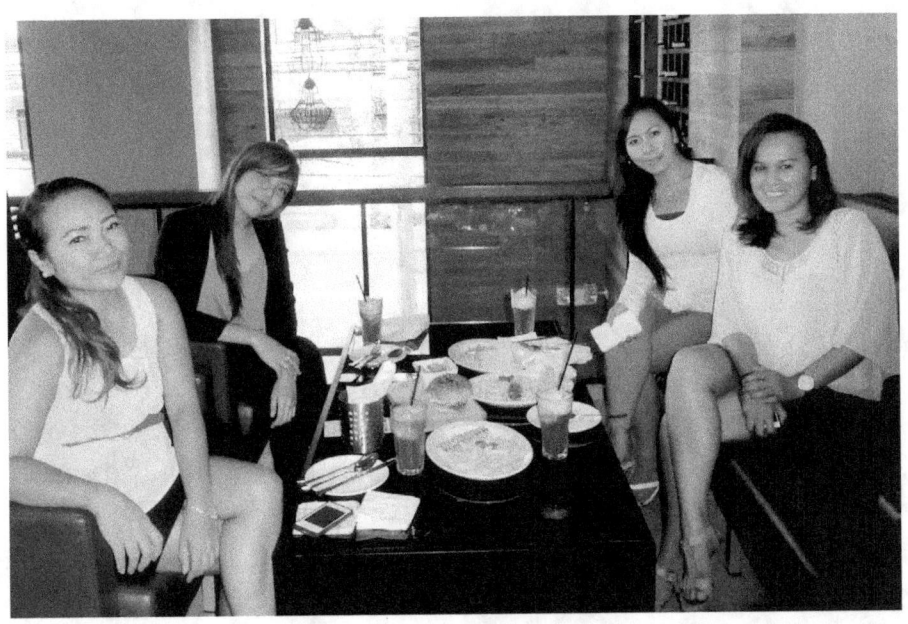

Brique is a good example of where you should take one of these beautiful 8's or 9s. Brique is an upscale Italian place that serves pasta, salmon and everything in between. I dropped about $20 bucks (1k pesos) and it was well worth the extra money. Cheap for us (Applebees back home is more expensive) but expensive enough to keep most poor Filipinos out, ala The Competition. This is where you go with a Beauty contestant, winner or not.

Tsim Sha Tsui (& Tea Bar)

Located in Cebu Business Park, Tsim Tsui is a Japanese eatery, upscale and very nice without breaking your wallet. Be aware that many Korean girls (Hi-So) like to hang out here, not just Filipinas. Korean girls are notoriously high-maintenance and, while more stunning than any other Asian locale, I'd much rather spend the night smiling with a 7 than put up with last minute resistance all night with a 9.

Anzani

They have the best steak in the Philippines and their wine bar is to die for. As a Mediterranean restaurant they are a bit pricey, but that's what is needed with a high quality girl. You want the perfect place for a romantic dinner. They also serve seafood (salmon), pasta and scallops but many other exotic foods too, like grilled crocodile.

I booked their cellar (downstairs) where many different wines were piled high right up to my waist! The in-house bread/tomato soup combo is also very good.

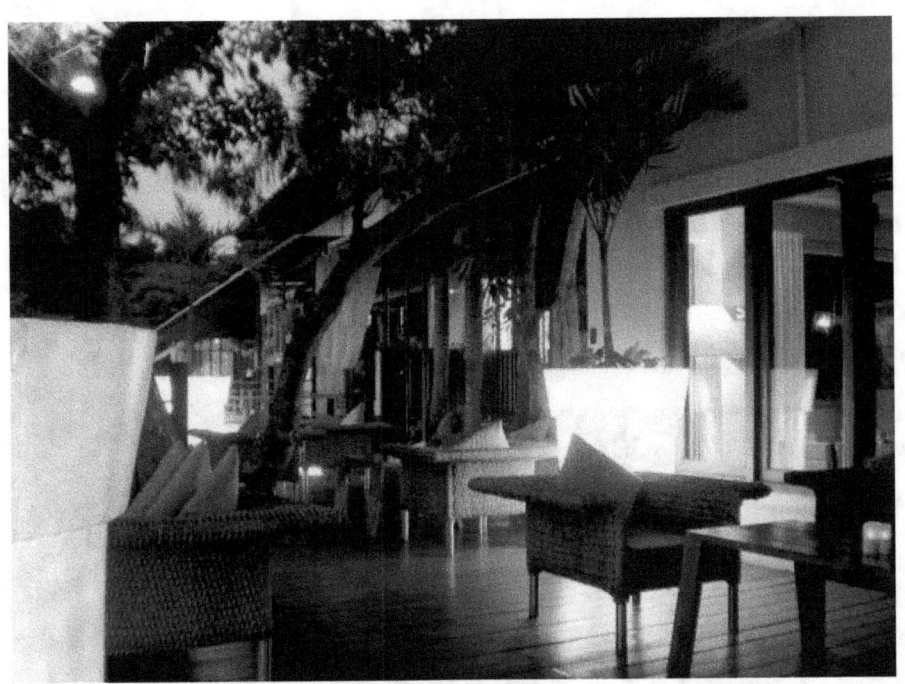

Costabella Island Resort

I took my beauty contest girl here and got the royal Emperor & Empress treatment. Two days seemed like two years in Paradise and I wish now that I had booked 4 days like I had originally planned. At $130/night it wasn't cheap, but this same experience would cost three times as much in the States for a white sandy beach, two large pools and a water level of 4 feet that extends quite a ways out before the deep end. Take your beauty queen out to collect seashells and starfish, or go parasailing.

Alternatively, you can take her to swim with whale sharks in Oslob city, about 3 hours south of Cebu. Bus tickets were 170 each way but it's an experience you cannot replicate in the West.

1500 pesos per hour seems like too short of a time but it really isn't when you consider the tide and waves. You can get quite close to them (though not allowed to touch unfortunately) *so bring an underwater camera if you can. You will wish you had!*

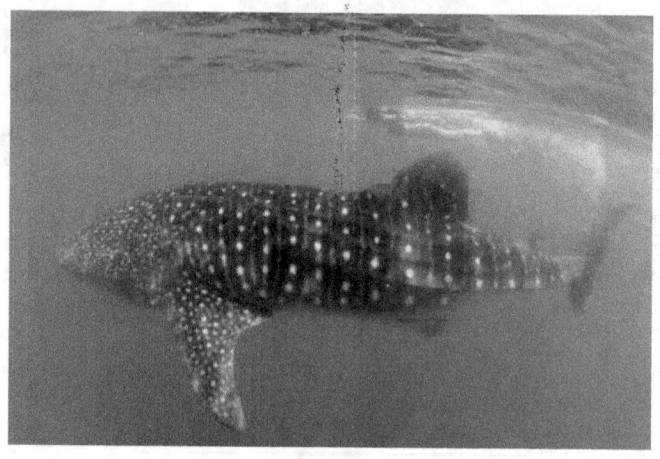

Chapter 4: 18 Year Olds

Age gap? None!

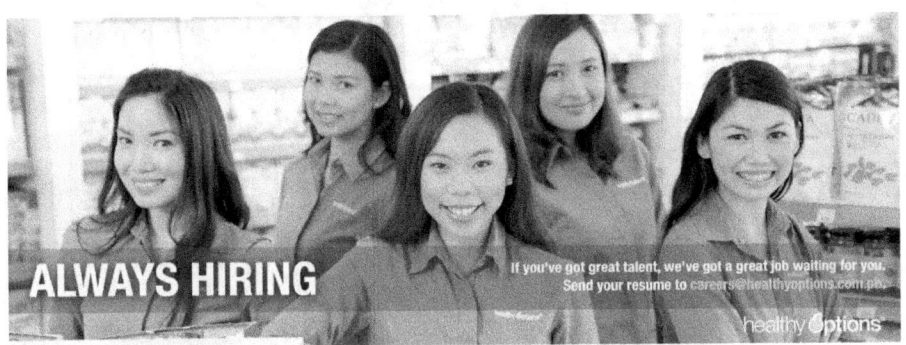

Which two are 18 years old?

I'll let you in on a little secret. Any of the above 6-7 range girls will swim naked with just about *anyone who looks stable and is nice to them.* All the sooner if he's a foreign nice guy. 'Nice Guy' just works in the Philippines. In Toronto, any of these cute little angels would call the police and label you a creepy stalker if you are 25 or above and hit on them in public.

Not in Asia. Here it's a whole different ballgame. No joke, girls here compete with each other for your affection. They know the score.

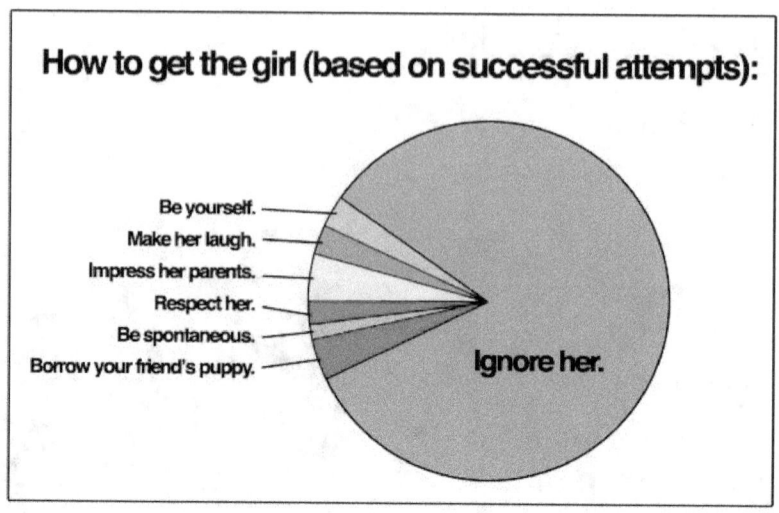

How to get the girl (based on successful attempts):

- Be yourself.
- Make her laugh.
- Impress her parents.
- Respect her.
- Be spontaneous.
- Borrow your friend's puppy.
- Ignore her.

The above picture illustrates how a guy gets the girl in the West. In the Philippines, you need to reverse this chart as Filipinas do not like being ignored. Ignoring her signals that you are not interested in her, ever, and are most likely banging other chicks. They do not play the psych games that Western women do so you do **not** need to 'figure them out psychologically' before proceeding to give them the privilege of your attention or finances.

Schedule Multiple Dates

Throw a lot of money around and you'll attract the wrong women who'll lie their panties off about their age. That said, 18 year old non-pros do come with a few challenges of their own that have nothing to do with money.

1.) Flake City. They're inexperienced and don't know responsibility (or your value)
2.) Difficult to isolate. Auntie Guardian of Lucy's virginity wants a free meal.
3.) Little darlings lie about age. A lot. Many own fake IDs.

There's a way around these problems, however.

Let's assume you are there for one week only for lack of funds or time or whatever. You wanna get in fast and get out fast as you don't have the luxury of a month long nymph splurge. But you also don't want to wait around a week or two to 'get to know' a girl before she drops the panties. What to do?

For starters you can weed out the time-wasters by scheduling **four dates a day** the first few days - ten dates total.

Hit the ground running.

A few girls will flake and I can guarantee 90% will be a half hour late because of traffic or other reasons.

Out of those ten dates you will snag a couple of hot mermaids to take to a nice hotel away from the family to do all kinds of kinky things with, in addition to:

- Snorkeling & Swimming with whale sharks
- Skinny dipping by moonlight
- Romantic dinner
- Seashell Collecting
- Jet Skiing

- Parasailing
- Whatever else comes up

If she busts your chops with drama you can kick her pimply butt out and replace her with another cute girl. It is here where a pipeline is like GOLD.

Don't Chicken Out

Don't make the mistake I made on my first trip to Cebu. For the first day or so I laid in bed as paralyzed as a paraplegic, suffering from self-imposed paralyzation by over-analyzation. Analyzing things to death.

I wanted to go home immediately where I felt 'safe' from all these drug cartels in Cebu and Davao (laughable!). The rest of the 2 weeks didn't amount to much more. So just go and have the time of your life and have as much sex as your body allows with the prettiest young thing in the bunch.

Like I said, if she throws down *any* drama then it is easy to replace her with one of the other Filipinas from the ten dates. She knows the score and that you have the upper hand.

I found that even with my average looks, I could hook up with smoking 18 and 19 year olds who were flattered beyond flattery that I wanted to treat them. Half of them viewed me as a rich foreigner who was about to sweep her and her family into the sky for a romp in my towering castle in the clouds. The other half found me 'fun and goofy' and said, 'Why not?'

Did I mind either outlook? Nope, and neither will you because you're going to show her the time of her life, one that she'll treasure forever.

And you will have an absolute blast doing it!

A Few Words of Wisdom on Dating 18 year olds

1.) Flakes - You mustn't fret over teenage chicks who flake in Manila or anywhere else because doing so lowers your perceived value. Young mermaids like these likely nurse fears of being seen with you and labeled a golddigger or pro. Cebu & Manila are gossip mills as it is, so promise a subtle location out of range of friends and family - like the Marco Polo.

Never allow her to introduce her parents or her siblings unless you want her attached to your side at all times. Her protective sister may even get suspicious and throw down drama ('What? You mean you don't even know his last name?')

2.) **Alcohol** - One sultry night in the New Orleans French Quarter I bought this girl, a dead ringer for Traci Lords, a drink. One random act of kindness, a hand grenade as I recall, and I was charged with 'contributing to the delinquency of a minor; a fifteen year old girl.

Avoid hard liquor with 18 year olds even in Asia if you can help it. Wine coolers are fine but avoid anything that sounds ominous (i.e. 'Hand Grenade', 'Antifreeze').

3.) **Get Her Alone** - This can be tricky as once the family finds out a rich stallion foreigner is interested in deflowering their precious Princess they will pull out all the stops to spy on you. Friends, too, may try to turn you into a frustrated gelding. Such 'friends' are the worst cockblockers in the world.

Get her alone. Gauge her interest in you by bouncing from McDonalds/Jollybee to another cafe, club or someplace quiet. Be the leader. Do not chase her. Do not allow her to lead. You decide where to go, when to leave, etc. Have an angle if it helps but never stay in the same spot all night unless you've business there.

4.) **Beware the Tears**

Filipinas wear their hearts on their sleeves and a few cry after making love. Heck many will cry *while making love* and this dupes a lot of western guys into falling hard for them.

Don't fall for it.

Filipina's flip feelings like a light switch and she'll be over you long before you are over her. Most women are like this. If you doubt this fact then have a listen to 'Women Know How to Carry On' by Waylon Jennings.

Filipinas here are gaming many, many more men than men are gaming women! Where her family is concerned there is so much more on the line than just a simple date.

5.) **Be Prepared!**

Where can one find the sexiest 18 year old in the Philippines? Anywhere! Trikes, cafes, markets, salons, SM Mall, college campuses.

The more important element here isn't them. It's you! You must be prepared at all hours because you can never predict when a sexy fertile young girl will pop up to talk to you. This took me by surprise because it never happened to me in Canada.

Whatever happens, never say, "Hold on while I jet to the john to fix my hair/brush my teeth/some other lame excuse" You must be prepared in advance for her arrival as a thief in the night.

You need to develop a sixth sense for when a girl just wants to rip a guy's clothes off. They do not care about your Ph.D in Neurology (boring!), they just want you to bang them next to a campfire after singing a guitar song. Are you prepped for that moment? What talent can you drop to get her spine tingling in a good way?

Always, always be prepared. Naturally she wants you to gel with her but there needs to be self-confidence on your part at the get-go. Girls can sense when a man expects to fill his needs by a certain girl but can also sense a faker. Self-doubt can be catastrophic.

Sexual Filters

The following will filter-out girls who are time-wasters or moochers and filter-in girls who are eager to bounce on your lap and sing their favorite songs to you in the bathtub.

Don't wait. Absolutely most important rule here. Establish sexual interest in the beginning. On my first trip to Davao I was with a 21 year old named Helen and I mistakenly believed I had to set the mood for this smoking Bond girl to drop her panties. You know - go slow, put on some Barry White mood music to candlelight and buy a kitten...

No No No! Touch early and often! They do not like mixed signals, so make your intentions clear or else she will get bored as quickly as a young kitten. Attention spans of moths!

- Ensure she sees you looking her sexy body over. Do not break eye contact.

- Joke with her about what she'd be like 'high' or 'drunk'.

- Dress sexual. Lookup her idols (singers, actors). How do they dress? Dance?

- Expose yourself. Go shirtless in your apt. It's hot! Filipinas worship white skin.

- Do not give a damn, son. If one girl rejects you, say 'Next' and go get another.

As an older guy in Cebu, you must light a sexual fire quickly. Any 18-20 year old is tired of the mind games teenage Pinoys (males) play and wants to have sex with an older white or black man <u>tonight</u>! She must look at you and think, "I wonder what sex position he likes?" A Filipina said to me in SM mall that this is what they think of when thin, nicely dressed 40-50yo guys walk by them in the Food Court. Not kidding. A few ballsy girls even mumble this if a foreigner and filipina walk by hand in hand.

At any rate you will either scare off the boring girls or massively turn on those who are into you. As a bonus you will not waste time with dim-witted Filipinas who don't know a good guy when they see one.

"A deception that elevates us is dearer than a host of low truths."
- Pushkin

Chapter 5: Red Flags, Green Flags

Better the devil you know than the devil you don't.

This means that it is often better to deal with someone you are familiar with and know, even if they are not ideal, than take a risk with an unknown person or thing.

Listed below are a few RED flags to watch out for if you desire a special (read: committed) relationship. Though I'd advise you to memorize these even if you're solely in it for the notch counts, because when it comes to green flags, what you do not know (Red Flags) can be catastrophic whether you are Krauser the Mack Daddy or just a guy looking for The One.

Legions of 'Superfriends'

Does she talk to other foreign guys? Tons do at CherryBlossoms and DateinAsia, but she'll never tell you. She could be 'servicing' them right after you which makes you the biggest Eskimo brother (read: chump) of all and unfortunately there's really no way to know unless you get a friend to hit on her.

If they are in fact 'real' friends, you have to surpass expectations. She's already glorified you, but you still want to seed future possibilities a dump be on the horizon.

If her friends despise you, they'll pit her against you and then you'll be nothing more than a wilted plant to all of them unless... you give her ammo to defend you with. Whatever the case may be, never, ever let her lay down the terms over and over like some demented feminist judge or she will walk all over you. Things like

- She takes forever to respond.
- Changes venue without asking you (to satisfy her superfriends)
- Doesn't stick up for you when her 'friend' gets sarcastic with you at the club.

Any of the above causes you to lose face, and in Asia, face is everything.

Lavish Backgrounds

Check those fancy hotel shots on her FB page and CB. Who took the picture? She claims to be a provincial 'simple' girl yet can afford to stay at a 4 star hotel in Boracay? An exchange of 'valuables' took place. The bouncy kind.

This does not only apply to 4-star hotels but *any* luxury item not normally seen in the Phils.

Meet the Parents

... or not?

It's said that any Filipina who does this is in all likelihood a good girl. I say there's a flipside to that dark coin in that she may be trying to play 'Leader of the Pack.

It won't mean much if you meet them or not if she goes Black Wolf on you. The problem is that if you let her play two-bit dictator then she's the one defining the nature and flow of the affair. She's now the leader, not you. Here's how it goes:

She says she'd be hurt if you don't meet Mommie Dearest. You say no, she cries, you give in and in one fell swoop elevates herself above the rest of the Filipinas you're screwing. Any other girls who find out that you 'Met the Family' will hesitate to bang you on general principles. Anywhere.

Contemplate this on the tree of woe for a moment as you chow down on Uncle Leo's freshly dead rooster. Hint: it means no more head for you, sailor.

Oh maybe a bone here and there, but now that The Family is around you'll get tables scraps since *she's* the leader and not you.

There's two ways out of such a mess. One is to go dark - full radio silence as though a UFO picked you up mid-bang with a hot teen in Borocay and never heard from again. This means moving somewhere else obviously.

The other is to play a kind of reverse-seduction meta-jerk game; the kind George Costanza played whenever he wanted to break it off but didn't have the guts to go through with it. Only in this game you act like a wild caveman who takes what he wishes, when he wishes.

Greet Mom and Dad with dirty palms. Swing mom around the kitchen. Open the oven. Steal cookies. Spank grandma Bessie as she walks by. Gulp down dad's pricey whiskey. Swipe the biggest meat. Complain it's burnt! When your girl serves you another, bend her over and spank her. Hit on her sister, cousin, aunt and great aunt. Hand them your business card in case they ever want to 'do lunch'.

Call her the next day to see if she's still interested in pursuing the 'relationship'. In the end, no matter how bad she wants something, your freedom is more important than her flighty feelings.

Tampo

Drop her if she exhibits 'Tampo' (passive-aggression) without a good reason. This is when something is wrong but they do not say why. Most Pinays think this is harmless but us Western guys want to retch every time a girl does this. It's a real deal breaker for men who aren't mind-readers (me) and worse when the girl is a stunner and the guy (me) doesn't have the balls to ditch her.

A friend's girl seduced her way into living with him and not long after, started tampo. She gave him the silent treatment for a whole week. With bitch shields at full strength, he begged her to tell him what was wrong at every place imaginable, following her around like some starving puppy suffering blue balls.

She gelded him because he was Nice Guy Eddie who refused to say no.

I blasted his balls with some red pill buckshot. Look, I'd said. You pack her bags outside the apartment and after that demand to know why she is so upset... or tell her to go to hell.

The next day she hands the apt key back to him in total silence and was never heard from again. Good riddance! The man suffered a few nights of full balls but come two months later he is thanking me for sparing his life from years of dark elf servitude. He's now back to banging 18 year olds.

DROP her the first time she does this. Just move on the next 99 girls in your phone. You are the prize, not her.

Money

Paying for dinner is one thing. Paying for cancer treatment for her sick dad is something else. But in the Phils how do you know her dad really has cancer? Or that he is sick at all?

Then there's her sick cow, her sick Auntie, her sick nephew who lives in the mountains with no phone service.

One very hot call center girl on DateinAsia almost succeeded in ripping me off to the tune of a hundred dollars. She begged me to buy the company's product so she could win a 'bag of rice' for her starving family. I called her bluff and rightfully so as later I found her to be a lying slut.

The Taker

Watch out for any Filipinas who consistently *take* but never *give*. It's generally a rarity in the Phils but we Western guys are so used to American women being such greedy harpies that we assume such behavior is normal the world over. Not so.

Things like,

- Asking you to treat their friends/family long before you've met them.
- Endless texting online but ignoring your req to meet them. (Validation junkie)
- Begging for pasaload requests (Goldigger)
- Saying they are coming to your place or the mall alone, but bring a friend or Auntie Hilda.

Russian guys know women like these. Ukraine, too, is filled to the brim with them. Men give. Women take. The exception is Filipinas but even they are only reacting to supply and demand. They've no choice to present themselves as anything but givers since so many women throw themselves at men here. Good, strong, stable men who aren't cheating dogs are hard to come by and they know it.

White Lies

Filipinas (as I have found them to be) are generally terrible, horrible, incompetent liars when they do decide to lie (which is often). Call them on it and show them proof that'd sway even the most corrupt judge in the world and watch as she issues one denial after another.

It isn't that they lie more than their American counterparts. It's that they lie with the face of a chocolate-faced kindergartener and think you're as dumb as she is.

"I've never done anything like this."
"We're not having sex tonight."
"I love you."
"My phone died unexpectedly..."
"I have a headache"

Ladyboy Conniseur

Never underestimate crazies. I thought it'd be easy-peasy to spot the ladyboy and avoid them. Then a 19yo girl named Thelma (yes, that was her name) from Cebu I enjoyed spending many a well-oiled night on the beach under moonlit nights introduced me to her ladyboy brother who worked in a salon in Cebu, right across the street from my regular barber shop! Drama ensued whenever haircut day came around. Avoid if possible or expect ten times the validation queen.

Suzie Two-Faced

Suzie, while an attractive, bone-inducing Filipina in her own right, cannot resist cutting down others in front of you when they're not there to defend themselves.

Friend or foe, doesn't matter but then she barely even knows *you*. What do you think she's going to do when you're not around? All the worse if she is cutting down her mother, father or siblings. Ditch her.

The Black Widow

File this one in the 'never asks you to use a condom' drawer, aka rawdogging. These are girls who are as fond of the black widow technique.

The technique is where they suddenly lock you in place with their legs just as you try to pull out. One 'gets away' and come a scant 9 months later she's got you by the balls if you didn't use Vasalgel.

Let me make a suggestion. If you encounter the Crazy Black Widow chick, DO NOT DELETE her number on your phone. A few months may breeze by when she calls out of nowhere and you get stuck in her web again. Just leave her number but change the name to Psycho, Black Widow or Crazy Cat Lady. This way you won't get duped into accepting her calls or texts when she tries to lure you into her trap once more.

The Mute Girl

Many Filipinas fall into this category on account of
shyness. Others do not. You can save yourself mind
melting boredom by taking note of her conversational level
before you spend money on her. The Mute Girl rarely
says two words no matter where you go about your
business in the Philippines. On Dating sites this usually
translates to 1-3 sentence messages. If this is the case,
expect the Silent Movie experience at:

Waterfalls.
Nightclubs.
Ziplines.
Kayaking.
Bars, Hotels, Pools...

She *does* speak English. She just doesn't like to talk.
Period. Other times it may be a case of incompatible
chemistry. With 18 year olds you need to constantly venue
skip, convo skip, liquor skip because they get bored as
quickly as toddlers. With 23 and up, there are a few things
you need to answer before she asks. Things like:

Do you do cool things? (Navy dolphin trainer who disarms
WWII bombs?)
Are you interesting? Well traveled?
Write novels? Shorts? Screenplays?
What's so different about you than other guys?
Can you simplify all this without coming off as an elitist
snob?

These are signs you may have a good girl on your hands. Moreover, you should not ever have to implicitly ask her, online or off, if she measures up to any of these qualities as they should be GLARINGLY obvious without you saying a word.

The Accountant

This girl has learned her lesson over handing money out like Skittles. Gambling and cock-fighting are huge in the Philippines and many a Pinoy has deeply rooted addictions and getting off the addiction is like getting off crack-cocaine.

When the well runs dry they'll seek out the most gullible chumps they can find, usually anyone that'll 'loan' them money without question. (Oh look, a rich foreign man!

The Accountant, though, doesn't loan out money. Period. She gives it on occasion but never for a case of Red Horse beer & cigs in a red-hot cockfighting contest in Manila. This is a girl you trust with your money.

But never credit cards.

The Cinderella Girl

This girl knows the score and her place. She cooks. She vacuums. She dusts. She wants your place clean and gets right to it without being asked because, let's face it, if she doesn't there are ninety-nine other sexy girls in Davao who will. She does this for you long after the initial meetup for the simple reason she wants to see you smile. She's a giver, not a taker.

When she cooks something you are the first to be seated and the first to eat. Her phone is off and so is any criticism. Then she asks you if you'd like your toenails clipped. Always say yes - evenly, all the way across.

The Accountable

"I'm getting my hair done today and a few other things," she tells you by text. Before you ask what 'other things', she tells you straight up the who, what, when and where and even the time she'll be back. She never turns her phone off while out.

The Good Girl

Never has sex on the first date. She's no virgin but even DiCaprio would give up at cracking that last minute resistance. Heated kissing, sure, but even that requires a soft tact and patience. By date three she'll gladly give it up since she knows temptation by other beauties roaming the Phils can be volcanic.

The Philosopher

Unlike 'Mute' girl, you can have long, interesting discussions on any topic. While not exactly Aristotle, she understands (or at least tries to) your metaphysical ramblings from studying Kant as an undergrad or your field study of mating tarantulas in the bayous of New Orleans, and even makes snide comments on Trevor's 'seriously disturbing personality disorder' during a sexually-distracting GTA5 session with you.

Unfortunately many 'smart' girls like this want to be the dominant one in the relationship. Same in Montreal.

The Museum Clerk

Like the young warrior who is asked by the chief to watch over his home while he is away in battle, your stuff is as good as safe. She won't raid your fridge without asking. She won't flip through your passport. She won't hire a hacker to break into your phone, email, or laptop. In fact she won't touch a thing you haven't given express permission for her to touch and doesn't ask the airport clerk or hotel concierge about your comings and goings. What's that verse in Proverbs about a woman's worth and rubies?

The Protector

She protects you and your wallet. Speaking Tagalog, she tells the cabbie not to even think of charging his 'special price' for foreigners. Same with buying anything really: real estate. Hotel prices. Market veggies. Whatever. She has your back and gives new meaning to the idea of a 'side piece'. Doc Holliday would be quite the jealous sixshooter.

The Great Communicator

This type of Filipina doesn't wait around for a small issue to evolve into a big, explosive issue. They have a six sense for such things.

Addictions, affairs, jealous friends, she can spot them all a thousand miles away at sea in stormy weather. Whether iceberg or not, expect her to bring it up for close inspection early rather than later. She wants no late-breaking hull breaches.

Chapter 6: Underage Girls

A Berliner, a New Yorker, and a Manilan were talking about the police in their respective cities. The Berliner says, "in Berlin, when a crime is committed, the police arrive in 5 minutes". The New Yorker replied "that's nothing. In New York, when a crime is committed, the police are on the spot in 3 minutes flat". The Manilan replied "in Manila, when a crime is committed, the police are already there."

Takeaway: Be careful. Some of these teens sting.

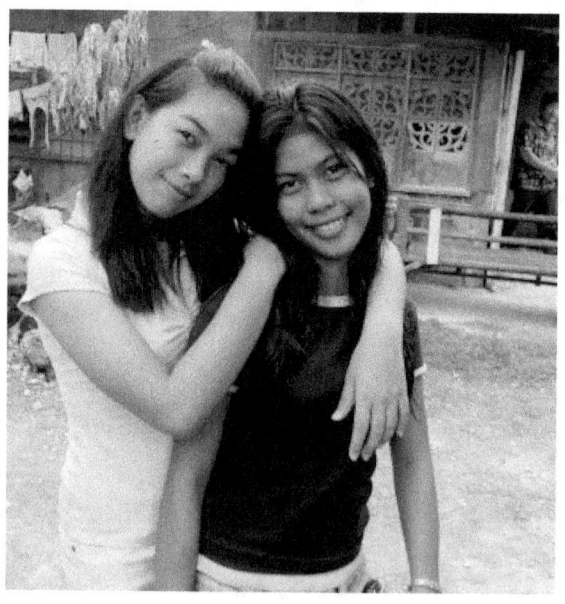

Which girl is 18?

If you picked the girl on the left as being 18 (violet shirt), you're wrong. If you picked the girl on the right, that's wrong too. They're 16 and 17, but you never doubted that at least one was 18, right?

They will tell you they are 18 if you ask them. Bar locations give guys a fake picture. They assume the girl has been carded and 'verified' by the bouncer. In all my travels it never mattered which city or mall I was in because they will lie to you about their age for a number of reasons. Status. Convenience. Free drinks or just plain mooch off of you. A good 20% of the girls I met in SM Malls across Cebu, Manila, Davao and Illigan weren't in fact legal to drink at all let alone have sex with.

If you're a western guy and get caught having sex with a girl under 18, you'll do serious time and when it's all finished do even more time in the USA on a double stretch since it is a federal crime for a U.S. resident to visit another country intending to have sex with a minor. Yes, it's double jeopardy, but U.S. politicians no longer care about the Constitution or a law-abider's rights either stateside or abroad. They want cold hard cash and nice headlines and banging 17yo girls abroad tickles their wallets like no other. It's an international racket.

Food Courts

Food courts and cinema and smoothie-type shops are where these teens hang out. If you're looking for 18 year olds though, you're better off hanging where the adults hang because they can verify her age. Her fellow teenage friends will lie for her at the Smoothie Shop. Count on it.

Picture yourself sitting down in the Food Court of any major mall in Cebu or Manila. You've unpacked your stuff back at the hotel - cologne, cash, suntan oil, passports - and now just want a little relaxation so you head on out for some R&R. Only as you start to read the paper outside an upscale cafe, two pony tailed pretties skip up to your table, uninvited.

Her: Hey! You're too handsome to eat all alone!

(You look them over. 21 you'd guess)

You: Wait, ah... um... where're you from darlin'?

Her: Tondo.

You: Tondo? Tondo... that's sounds like a nice place.

Forget for a moment that Tondo is Asia's equivalent to Mogadishu and ask yourself if you have the balls to ward off these vampires. Most expats don't and it's surprising since all it takes is just one word: No.

No No No. Tell her and her little succubus friend to bugger off.

Do not be Mr. Nice Guy. Do not be Clark Kent. Be a rude foreign bastard if your gut even suspects they are underage because most likely they are and you are being setup for a sting.

It is hard enough to tell even in broad daylight who is 17 or 18 or 21 and harder still at night. Mannerisms usually give the age away with Western girls but here, Pinays are a different breed than your average U.S.-born Filipina. They lure thirsty foreign men better than Mae West and could put Cleopatra to shame in a makeup contest. The only real way to lift the veil is to ask for ID.

It works but you must be **vigilant** about asking for it up front and *not when you've already brought her back* to your hotel room. By then it is far too late.

It is against the law to be in a hotel room with a minor, even if there is no sex, unless the girl is a relative. You step one foot into that room and you're under arrest, buddy.

A new Cebu city ordinance requires hotels to report underage girls entering their premises or risk serious fines and closure. Not only are the cops watching, but hotel employees are too. They're all looking to squeeze cash from you so don't think just because you help pay the salaries of hotel employees that they'll be on your side.

Entrapment

Entrapment is huge in the Phils. But let's say you ignore your gut-check and invite her over anyway because of a few smart things she said that made you believe she's older than she appears. Here's what will usually happen:

You'll go two minutes in your posh Marco Polo hotel room with sexy little Tawny when she'll ask to use the phone.

That's so she can invite the other girl over. Then there's a knock at the door, but it isn't her friend. Before you can even answer it, the cops (PNP) storm in with M16's pointed at your head and start screaming in that awful Tagalog dialect. Then the girl conveniently shows her birth certificate that bears her true age: 17.

17!

Alice Cooper never wrote a song about banging 17 years olds. I think I know why.

The police then get you to pay as much as you can get from your ATM. $2000 clams or more. One news report said a fellow was scared to death as they put the M16 to his head and threatened to kill him if he so much as breathed a word of it to anybody.

Another scam involved a fellow Canadian from Montreal who'd just arrived in Manila. He settled in, unpacked, went out for a walk to get some fresh air and a smoke and met up with a group of young teens shooting the breeze. Being a blabbermouth, he ends up blabbing the name of his hotel. When he returns, the police are there at his room who tell him, "You've been with underage girl".

He denies it up and down. Yells. Swears.

Then the girl comes in and says "That's the one officer..." pointing directly at him. The police tell him he has to come with them to the police station. So he went and they had a table out in front of the station on Roxas Blvd where the girl's "mother" was sitting. He knew it wasn't the mother, but the police asked how much he could afford to pay this so-called "mother" or they would lock him up. He paid quickly - to the tune of $500.

It is worth noting that many of these setups and scams occur in the usual hangouts: Red light districts or streets where foreigners of a certain depravity gather: Ermita, P. Burgos, Angeles City. Avoiding these places significantly reduces your chances of such an encounter.

Cinemas and Pools

Swimming and cinema trips with your girlfriend's niece must be done WITH THE GIRLFRIEND or someone else who qualifies as a relative. Should you be in a situation where you are left to supervise any child due to the guardian not being present, you must explain and refuse to undertake such a supervisory role. The same applies to any house or method of travel, shopping or restaurants since all it takes is some broke Pinoy to suspect you are with a child illegally and tail can be locked up for a long time.

In the Philippines, you are considered guilty until proven otherwise by a court of law.

Chapter 7 Test Your Filipina's Loyalty

There are two (effective) ways to test a Filipina's loyalty. One way is ethical and the other, not so ethical.

<u>The Ethical Way</u>

How I tested one girl's loyalty.

I decided to visit a friend in Dumaguete as a litmus test of sorts, but only gave my girlfriend, Angel, *juuuust* enough info to tickle her curiosity. I *did not* tell her the trip was only to swap business advice over beers with this friend of mine. For all she knew, I was building three brothels next to a cockfighting arena with intentions of being the grandest pimp daddy in the Phils.

I just said, "Seeing a friend." Nothing more. Nothing less. The expression on her face told me she suspected I was about to bang multiple women on the beach while sipping margaritas like her previous Pinoy boyfriend had a few months prior. He'd broken the dear girl's heart, she'd said, but I'd had a pretty clean streak and now she was suspicious.

If my girl had breathed a word of protest then that's exactly how I would've ended up. Margaritas and up to my neck in hot girls. A bonus was that I knew she had saved money (she was half-Chinese and very good at it). She wasn't rich or even upper-class, but certainly had enough for a plane ticket to Dumaguete.

"Meet me there," I told her. I didn't ask. I didn't offer to pay for it. I just said meet me there. No explanation other than "It'll be the experience of a lifetime."

She flew in and I couldn't have been happier to pay for her return trip plus the amount she spent flying in. We had a blast. I took her to things she never could have afforded on her own and the look on her face every night was PRICELESS.

This was a major deal and I realize your average provincial girl may not have the funds to pull off something of this caliber, but there are other ways.

- Ask her to take pictures of the Jun n' Dell Apartment complex you're considering staying at

- Ask her to talk to the Front Desk clerk at the Marco Polo. Do they allow pets?

- Ask her to go to a free convention and take pics. If she says 'Google it', dump her.

- Ask her to sample a high end restaurant (Brisq) with her mom or auntie (your treat) before you arrive. Pay someone who works there to scope her out. Is she with family or some Pinoy she's banging on the side?

The point here is to watch what women DO, not what they SAY. You have to remember that most Filipinos operate on a moment-to-moment basis. Nothing beyond their immediate needs and desires even enter their mind.

The Unethical Way

Now for the Dark stuff. As long as you don't mind venturing into shady territory, there is in fact a foolproof way to find out if your Filipina girl is cheating on you.

Ready?

Buy her a cheap Android phone. Not too cheap, as you want her to use it every day, but cheap enough for the job. A Moto G fits the bill nicely and can be had for under a $100. Then, ethics aside, you install a keylogger.

Get a P.I to do it if you lack the technical prowess. Plenty of private eyes do in the Phils.

Whoa... wait. What's a keylogger?

Keyloggers are spyware that record all conversations - text, emails, etc. - so that everything typed gets recorded. Dozens of top shelf keyloggers exist for parents who want to keep their kids from dealing drugs, joining gangs, spraying graffiti, etc., and for that purpose it's really a godsend because most kids have never heard of them. For all others, well, it's shady as it's mostly used by divorce-seeking wives who *want* the hubby to stray so they have a reason to leave.

You alone have to decide if breaking your ethics for a couple of weeks to find out the trustworthiness of a filipina is worth it. Some say yes. Some no. Is a keylogger worth it if it prevents a future heartbreak and a divorce-rape? You better believe it. Better to discover her infidelities now than after the wedding.

You can be sure if the suspicion was on the other foot and you were the one traveling to and fro, she would not hesitate to install one on *your* phone given the opportunity. Do likewise but know that absolute power corrupts absolutely, so when the two week test is over, pull the plug.

Resist the urge to send her spiraling down into a shark tank the way Stromberg did to his lover in The Spy Who Loved Me.

Chapter 8: Where To Find 'Good Girls'

Sooo you want to find a good girl and settle down. Maybe sweet-talk a nice provincial girl into marrying you who:

- Does not sleep around.
- Cooks & cleans without bitching.
- Provides sex without asking.

In short, a girl who feeds you, bangs you, and shuts up. We can also add 'religious' to it, but be careful no to go *too* religious. Example.

A friend of mine, Barry, was raised in a conservative denomination and had himself a little porn problem in the marriage. It wasn't a problem for him but the wife disapproved. She divorced him over it.

(She'd have probably divorced him anyway, but this made for a convenient scapegoat)

He never hit her. He never cheated. He never gambled. He never drank or robbed anyone. The poor guy had been financially supportive of her for eons and loved his kids dearly, always putting them first before anything else.

"Either the porn goes or I go," she'd told him. She refused blowjobs and handjobs. Missionary only because her whoring youth was 'all behind her now'. She went and so did he. Lickety split.

Avoid such a woman like the Black Plague.

In the event you suspect you're with a woman like the above but don't have the brass balls to break her heart -- call up the cavalry. Ask the females of your family to judge your future bride. I can think of no other time when any of my own female relatives will look out for my best interests at heart. As a bonus these women will test for any incompatibility to themselves, because the last thing they want is another bitchy old crone to deal with whenever the Lake O' The Pines Family Reunion comes up.

The Where

Asia, mostly, as you'd have a better chance at winning the lottery than scoring a 'good girl' in the West, Australia or the UK. The other choices are:

1. Vietnam
2. Philippines
3. China
4. Thailand
5. Eastern Europe/Russia

For the Philippines I'd target laid back conservative cities like Dumaguete, Iiolo City and Davao and avoid Angeles City (monger central), Cebu (party girl central) and Manila (scammer central). If notch counts with 18 year olds are your only goal then by all means hit Cebu hard and pipeline heavy. If on the other hand you want a good girl to start a family with, these places are terribly sub-optimal for this goal.

For a good girl, you want quiet, out-of-the-way places that haven't been plagued by Western feminism or female careerism and all the hamster-entitlement-mentality that comes with. You want good mother material. A girl who had a great relationship with her father.

Stable households is what you should aim for; families that stick together like glue. No single moms, divorcees, mental cases, gambling addicts, dope dealers. Inspect that household like you were adopting a stray cat for your little girl. Check the history, the gums, the teeth, test for immune-system diseases, every little thing because better someone else suffer a broken heart than you.

Certainly a poor provincial girl needs care in this broken world too, but let another man go through the hell that comes with molding her into a responsible woman. Let some other guy deal with a drama queen who throws a fit because you refuse to take her to the lake.

Good Girl vs. Bad Girl Signs

A few more Red/Green flags

Good:

- Cooks for you at your place and hers. Pampers you like a King.

- Attends church regularly. Prays *outside* of church.
- Feminine features. Feminine face/figure. No 'carousel' stare.
- No Tattoos.
- Never disagrees with you in front of her family or your friends.
- Smiles with a pleasant attitude

Bad:

- Calls often. Where are you? Who're you with? (tough one for Filipinas. YMMV)
- Bank/Accounting position. Money ballbuster.
- 100 Facebook friends, all married except her.
- Hides a kid with Auntie in the mountains.
- Flashes tits on webcam on the first session.
- Bangs on first date (varies).
- Was a cheerleader or dancer (stripper).
- Wants to open a 'business' in the Phils with *you* as financier.
- Pressures to 'get married' after 3 months. Lots of Filipinas do this. Just be careful.
- Divorced

First Time Dates:

- **Holding hands**. Even if the first date is small coffee talk at Starbucks, if your Filipina withdraws her hand after a you briefly touch it... ditch her. Don't waste money on further dates, drinks, or ice cream cones because at this point she's signaled she's a big waste of time and doesn't care for your affection, only your money.

- **Crowded clubs**. We all know how crowded busy clubs can get. Restaurants too. If she doesn't want to sit next to you... ditch her. Princess thinks sitting next to you hurts her social status.

- **Walks Ahead**. A consistent 3 or more paces ahead of you at parks, streets, fairs, malls signals Mother Superior attitude... ditch her. She's got a massive superiority complex. I dated a Toronto woman who did this constantly until I finally broke it off. Avoid!

- **Horse Freak**. Any fascination with horses (tattoos, plates, statues, china), ditch her and double-check your condoms for pinholes. She's as mental as Quint was in Jaws, and at least he was entertaining. Something about 'taming' the wild stallion, never mind that the boat is on fire.

- **Won't Kiss**. Many dark-skinned girls feel inferior to white foreign guys so this can simply be due to shyness. She doesn't feel worthy. Plus, bad logistics can hinder a first date kiss leading you to think she doesn't like you. For Filipinas this usually coincides with giggles as they turn away. That's okay. As long as she doesn't act like western women (recoil in horror) then keep pressuring her to reciprocate and break down that wall.

- **Smartphone Addiction**. If a girl fidgets with her phone when a group of your closest friends are having a conversation instead of joining in, or at least listening, she's lost something of her humanity to her precious phone. Ditch her. It gets worse from here on out.

- **Manly Voice** - Most Filipinas love to sing. The ones that don't are smokers who sound like Marge's sisters Patty & Selma, the MacGyver nuts (no offense to MacGyver!).

Generally speaking, 'good' girls and 'grey area' girls prop us up even if we botch the date. At an Italian joint I had a cute 23yo girl I was into sit at 90 degrees instead of across from me so she could enact that all-important first touch (locking fingers) without having to *strrrretch* across the table.

She could sense how nervous I was and that nervousness made any flirtation on my part seem forced and unnatural, so she made it easier. We had sex later that night.

'Bad Girls' do not prop us up in the States and the Philippines are no exception. They tear us down to their level so they can feel like Mother Superior at the ready so as to whack you with her ruler when you get out of line. Intellectual conversation does not help. Touching does not help (it's too 'forward' in her mind). Any sexual tension is destroyed unless you're Leonardo Di Caprio.

Proofing a Good Girl

One test I like to give a girl who seems 'too good to be true' is to put her in a situation where she has to pick between me and her family, such as taking care of grandpa instead of going out to the Alcohology nightclub on Friday night. If she puts other's needs ahead of her own, that is a green light to something more serious.

For the foreigner who gets how flirtatious these filipinas really are, you must ask yourself what your goals are prior to visiting Asia:

Do you simply want notch counts?
Do you want a long-term girl?
Does she add to your life (value) or take it away?

When you see the habits of the average expat who escapes the west who is:

- glad to get a smile
- glad to get affection
- glad to make out with an 18 year old (whom he'll marry the next day)
- glad to bang on first date
- glad to have sex twice a day

Reality will hit you when you figure out the smoking 18 year old teenager with the Bond girl legs and blowjob skill is just another Filipina teen in a bag of skin. She's a hollow log. An empty potion bottle. You can raise the bar and aim for 9.5 Bond chicks but in the end they are women who entice you to wander around in a fog if they sense you're aimless. Then they want power over you and your business and they are very very good at extracting intel from you. Be careful.

Steinbeck, who wrote 'King Arthur and his Noble Knights', shed some light on this power trip women seem fond of. In one chapter, a young Lancelot licking his wounds, is trained by a frail old woman-in-hiding who grew up wanting to be a knight, much to the chagrin of her traditional father. She recants how once in a forest glade, she killed another knight in a fair fight but fled and hid away her knightly things to save her life and her father's reputation. After a lengthy sermon on what it means to be a 'just knight', Lancelot, still full of questions, asks what it is that all women want. She said,

"Power over a man. At any cost. Nothing else comes close."

You need a psychological connection and not just nipple engagement to be satisfied with yourself - i.e. the source of happiness for any man; a girl who has many other skillsets that go beyond sex fills this niche nicely. Beach bar owners, for example, know the score and want to return home after a long day and be excited to see sex *and* a great mind. Not just a bar whore.

Let's say you...

- Find a cute girl at an upscale cafe. A seven.
- Sleep with her.
- Want to keep her around but do not quite hear wedding bells.

Give her the 'Nice Guy' test. Show her a little niceness and watch her reaction. Western women (and Canadian women especially) will view such niceness as weakness. Toxic women who like bad boys and 'making a scene' fall into this category. Goldiggers too. Does your kindness green light further money requests?

If she rewards/likes your kindness in turn, she's a possible keeper. A good girl.

Before you marry her though you should find out what she likes to read. Story of O, 50 Shades = Bad. Jan Karon, Anita Shreve = Good. Does she like Christian rock or Justin Bieber?

Study her browser history.

Live with her for 1 year.

Warn her what your boundaries are and if she crosses them she can expect a swift kick to the curb.

Make a list of your needs, desires (sexual) and things you will never tolerate.

You need to train your girl how to love you and take care of your needs. So if she's agreeable to authority and your lessons, you're more likely to have the beautiful creature you've always dreamed of.

When to Hire a PI

Suspicious Motives

- Hypocrisy; she busts your hide for going out to Alcohology to get smashed but then does the same the following weekend.
- Has more male friends than you.
- New friends who work in a bar
- New tattoos; doesn't care what you think.
- Disappears/Won't return your calls (she's banging someone else)

PI Worthy Actions

- Encrypts her phone, keeps the password from you
- Applies for a credit card without asking you first
- Won't let you use her laptop. Ever.
- Mysterious bank withdrawals

Chapter 9: Cool Stuff That Didn't Fit Anywhere Else

What follows are a few scattered pearls that didn't quite fit in previous chapters. Mostly, I repeat myself. But some things need repeating because the brain will remember things said three times.

<u>Be Picky</u>

Be picky and aim high! That is, never settle for second best in the Phils or anywhere else because the next day after bedding that 5, an 8 will show up and ask you out. This happened to me when I first came to Asia. I settled far, far too low: a marketplace girl who looked 'average'. Anyway, it's a lot easier to say no when you already have an 8, so ask someone out that you perceive to be 'out of your league'. You may just surprise yourself.

If I could go back in time and give myself one piece of advice, it'd be this: Always go for the prettiest, sexiest, come-hither little thing you've ever laid eyes on. Do not settle for second best. She will say yes because you had the balls to ask despite your average looks.

In Toronto: "Haha! I can't believe that knuckle-dragger thinks he can get a date with me. Me! I feel all icky looking at him. Oh god he's looking at me again. Like, gross me green."

In Philippines: "Oh my god, that handsome man is staring at me! Me! Will he ask me out? What do I say? oh god here he comes! I think I'm gonna faint... "

Most girls in my native Canada as well as the USA do not approach a guy. That's a fact of life. They simply can't unless they're coked up on drugs, alcohol or other external stimulants that lower inhibitions (Montreal being the exception). Yet they are suffering inside with the urge to screw and if you don't approach then some clown will get the tail and you won't.

In the Phils many ladyboys and scammers and pros will approach you as soon as they see you. They figure you're rich. Super rich. Trump rich. How do you know a pro from a regular girl? It's a hard thing to discern. You'll probably bed a prostitute without knowing it till morning. Don't sweat it. Just give her a few pesos and chalk it up to experience. But whatever happens you musn't let yourself think these are Western Girls. Far from it.

Go Where Stunners Hang Out

My advice: pick the prettiest girl in the mall. That hot 21 year old in the jewelry shop with emerald eyes won't ask herself out. Go up, strike up a convo about some ridiculous thing, bad earrings or something, broken necklace, sneakers. Ask ridiculous questions and get so clown-funny that you make her laugh. This works in Asia. Not in the west (though do make her look busy since the bosses tend to frown on flirting while at work). When she settles down you can hand her your number business card.

If you do not bang that pretty little emerald-eyed beauty, someone else will! So go where the stunners hang out.

Victoria's Secret

Penshoppe

Bath & Body Works

HealthFoods

Disclaimer: Don't overdo the hand-the-number-out technique in SM Malls in the Philippines. Word spreads like wildfire and many a player have been milking this method for years. Not to say it doesn't work *at all* anymore. No, no. It's simply less effective now.

I had one girl, a smoking 8.5 with Victoria's Secret legs, tell me the date was off when she saw me flirting with other 18yo girls in neighboring shops. I asked why this should bother her. She said, "After seeing that I didn't feel 'special' no more."

Golddiggers

There's no way around it. Spend some time banging around the Phils and you'll run into a WildWest style golddigger. She's shadowy. She's flirtatious (phone sex voice). She's deadly. They're in every city and you cannot escape them. Luckily they will try and milk you early on so as not to waste time before moving on to the next chump on You Bet Your Wallet.

Show her no mercy. Be the mindless putz she thinks you are. You aren't of course, but don't let *her* know that. So sell her what she wants: The Gold. Tell her you're an up n' coming Western novelist with several cowboy romance novels to your name who just signed a 'large figure deal' with Harlequin to pen 10 novels over the next 7 years. (If you want to be really devious you could buy images on istock and pay some kid on fiver to whip up a fake novel cover and email them to her.).

By the time she figures out that your penned novels are as worthless as tumbleweeds in a six-shooting midget's bedroom, you've long since left but left that wet crevess between her legs red and rawhide. The trick is to bang quick and fast and dirty and get out of Dodge before the shooting starts.

Be Direct

Filipinas hate indecisiveness and fake confidence the same as Russian girls do. They sense it if you try to pull the wool over their eyes, same with the natural world where foxes try to outsmart their prey. Your eye movement and body language also betray you in ways you cannot begin to imagine because you're so used to trying to fake it till you make it in the good ole USA. Therefore go into any approach with the following in mind:

1. Never fear letting them know you're interested in sex.

2. Never say you're 'sorry' for it. You have testicles that produce testosterone. Never apologize for this.

3. Be there. No matter if you fear a terrorist attack, UFO invasion or an army of T-1000 Terminators showing up... just be there. Success in writing, women, wine tasting, whatever, comes from being there consistently day to day, hour to hour, and putting in the effort. Craft, like game, evolves by trial and error, not by being absent.

4.) Don't give a damn, Scarlet. Just don't. Do not care if she says no or blows you off. It's a numbers game and the next 7 girls behind her would love to be with you at the venue of your choice. You'll see!

Chapter 10: Don't Wait. Go Now.

In the USA, the system punishes the higher earner. In the Philippines & Thailand, the system rewards the higher earner.

In light of this you should buy that ticket for the Philippines or Thailand now, not later.

Most men never do. They put it off for 6 months until another, more easily accessible dream surfaces that still resides in the 'safe zone' dictated by Chase bank or their whip-wielding Drow elf wives.

They buy a Camaro or Accord or Harley thinking it'll heal their broken hearts and feminist-scarred minds. Black Mica w/ moonroof and Bose system with glow lights, that'll do the trick, they think. A new fire pit for the living room. Guys love fire pits. So do I. The way the fire dances along a girl's naked skin to induce a primal love making session - nothing else on this earth can compare. It often leads to rough sex.

But some men use these things as an excuse to not take a chance. They buy toys, eat Cheetos, and buy cheap wine to numb the pain and never escape the system that rewards bad female behavior and punishes male success. They exchange liberty for a little pleasure up until the court assigns the fire pit to the ex and new boyfriend who plan to celebrate the festivus over champagne.

Listen. I collapsed at work three months before I left the West and it turned out to be the biggest wake-up call of my life. This happened in my 40s and I erroneously assumed that since I exercised, I was immune to stress.

I ate healthy. I spent 3 days a week in a Tae Kwon Do class. I ran.

But the more stress I took from my hyper-critical warpig boss, the more I turned the cheek, the more I played it safe, the more crap I ate from Taco Bell - the higher my chances of collapsing into an early grave. When my doctor told me I had a year to live I quickly glanced at the wall calendar to check if it was April 1st.

He wasn't kidding. Exercise or not, working for a fiery dragon lady was like being force-fed a little bit of mercury each day. That is just what she wants. Power over a man, at any cost.

Stress kills. Dominant women kill.

The slow chipping away at one's soul in the form of nagging, criticism, and putdowns will wear down any ambition and self-confidence you have built up. Your soul and body are linked. I do not care what the atheists say, I've experienced it.

You will get diabetes, strokes, panic attacks, Alzheimer's and a host of other parasitical problems that rob your future and your past and kill the here and now that rightfully belongs to you and you alone. Most of these stem from worry and anger, which can be managed, certainly, but when combined with a bad woman it's like a bulky wagon pulling jars of nitroglycerine over a rocky desert passage. Sooner or later... kaboom.

They also stem from not having any authority in your life. No power. Not having your say. No domain. This isn't the way God intended it. God wants *you* to be the boss. So do not be a pushover. Do not procrastinate.

Staying in the West where it is 'safe' instead of traveling overseas is like a raccoon walking into a cage, eating the bait egg and staying there when the trap fails in hopes he'll get another egg that isn't so rotten. Do not work for an egg given by a raccoon-faced woman manager. Do not trade your heart for cash. Do not sell your soul for high-risk no-reward safety in the West.

Life in the West is horribly unfair to men. It's a fact. If life was fair, you'd be happily married to that pretty girl from sixth grade because you swiped that evil spiked caterpillar off her shirt when she cried out for help.

But that's not the case is it.

You realize that something is wrong because the whole western system is wired to defeat strong and courageous men. Western women pull the strings in this matrix. Normal men get ruined. Lose everything. You can sleep with a sexy girl and wake up to a police 'knock and talk' where they accuse you of rape and perversion and yell "You're a creep!" as they slap the cuffs on and all while Nelly speeds across town to bang the next chump right into a jail cell.

Pregnant by some guy in the club stall? You get to pay child support because the judges and activists love good headlines, justice be damned. These kind of women are like the little trained minions of Sauron. They Do Not Share Power.

Solution:

Leave that toxic environment behind and go out and chase sunshine, surf and young pussy in Asia. Remember this: the pain of regret is far worse than the pain of rejection, and if you stay in the west you give them more power. Leave now and go get yours.

You never know when the black caddy will come calling.

May God bless and keep you on your journey!